Table of Content

Tasty KETO

recipes for beautiful

skin and body

By

Tina K. Bing

Introduction

Ketogenic diet is the most popular and nowadays mostly discussed diet for weight loss. Scientists have recently published all new research proving the benefits of an unusual diet which includes a process that forces the body to get energy from fat rather than carbohydrates.

In research, it is shown that consuming a large amount of fat, a moderate amount of protein and a small amount of carbohydrates can have positive impacts on health:

- Lower cholesterol level
- Lose excess weight;
- Lower blood sugar;
- Increase energy potential.

Have you ever wondered how much the foods that you eat can affect the condition of your skin? There are many theories linking an unhealthy diet to various skin problems.

How is the low-carb diet and skin condition related? In the ketogenic diet, the ingredients that negatively affect the skin of the face are mostly excluded.

If we follow the statement that beauty comes from within, it is necessary to take into account the fact that a healthy food will positively influence our skin, and unhealthy food will create problems, in some cases - chronic. Some foods consumed in excess and for a long time can provoke negative skin changes: acne, wrinkles, eczema, and so on.

Refined carbohydrates

While talking about refined carbohydrates, we usually refer to sweets, cakes and other popular products that do not contain important nutrients, such as B vitamins, fiber, and iron but these products are rich in white flour and sugar. So when we eat these in large quantities, they increase the production of androgens. Androgen, a kind of male hormone, which stimulates the activity of the sebaceous glands and consequently, the sebaceous glands produce more sebum than usual. Well, we all know that excess sebum clogs the pores, leading to acne.

Sugar

The problem of the effect of sugar on the body is quite complex, and it starts with a process called glycolysis. During glycolysis, sugar in the blood joins the proteins and prevents their normal functioning. Collagen is an important component of the skin which contains about 40% of the body's protein. When the collagen fibers are exposed to sugar, they lose elasticity due to glycolysis. The negative impact on the skin can be seen severely and its premature aging.

Also, sugar is associated with various problems of digestion, which, in the end, not only harms our health but also affects our skin badly.

Salted products

Nobody argues that salty snacks are incredibly delicious. But it is worth thinking a bit before sitting relaxed in front of the TV with a big bowl of chips, as excess sodium leads to the same consequences as foods rich in saturated fats do. Salt retains fluid in the skin cells, leading to swelling of the tissues and loss of elasticity.

Fats

You should know that when we eat excess sugar and refined carbohydrates, the body turns them into fats. It is necessary to understand that not all fats are useful for our health, and those obtained from sugar are not obviously the best of them. How can this be related to skin problems? Well, that's a pretty simple question. First of all, our skin needs oxygen to maintain its health. Oxygen actually facilitates the production of collagen, elastin and other vital elements. On the other hand, fats reduce the amount of oxygen that enters into the cells of the skin. In addition, sugar blocks the release of linoleic acid, which is indispensable for the body and this causes dermatological problems.

Dairy

Many studies have shown that dairy products can adversely affect the condition of the skin. It was found that all dairy products (except yogurt) and especially milk, increase the likelihood of skin ailments. Many healthy recipes can be created with yogurt, and that is why it is becoming more popular. It can also be used as an ingredient in your home remedies for beautiful skin.

Carbonated drinks and caffeine

You have already heard that maintaining a balanced blood glucose level is necessary to have a beautiful skin. Soda is rich in sugar, artificial sweeteners, and caffeine. So these drinks have every chance to cause some skin problems such as acne or wrinkles.

In addition, caffeine increases excitability, which means a predisposition to stress. When you are experiencing stressful moments, your skin loses blood and oxygen, which makes it lifeless. So if you want to have a beautiful skin and actually care about the skin, caffeine is a undesirable no for you.

Alcohol

Long gone are those days when alcoholic cocktails were considered as the best way to cheer up. There is no doubt that moderate consumption of alcohol can be beneficial to health, but increased doses of booze entail some serious side effects. If it is important for you to maintain a radiant appearance, remember that alcohol dehydrates the skin, as sodium does. Alcohol also dilates the blood vessels until they lose tonus, causing harmful effects on the skin. Alcohol is also responsible for broken capillaries, wrinkles, and the development of acne in the skin. If you are always worried about how to have a beautiful skin, follow the simple tip and cut down your alcohol consumption.

Spices

If you are prone to face reddening, then it can be heat or spicy food. Spices increase blood flow and lead to an expansion of the visible blood vessels on the face.

So, if you want to look younger, impress people around you with glowing healthy skin, make sure that you have the right set of ingredients in your diet. Everything that is delicious in your kitchen will not necessarily bring grace to your face.

Ingredients you should consume to have flawless body and skin:

• Fermented milk products of high-fat content

• Eggs;

• Meat (minced meat, steaks, meat for suppression, pieces of fillet, etc.);

• Fish (preferably greasy) and seafood;

• Hard cheeses (try to choose cheeses with a minimum amount of carbohydrates);

• Oils (creamy, unrefined vegetable, coconut);

• Mushrooms;

• Vegetables rich in fiber;

• Cabbage (white, colored, Brussels, etc.);

• Other vegetables that grow above the ground;

• Nuts, nut pastes;

• Avocado;

• Pumpkin seeds;

• Salad leaves.

In the minimum quantity are allowed:

• Dark, bitter chocolate with a maximum content of cocoa and a minimum of sugar;

• Raw root crops, vegetables, fruits not thermally processed;

• Tea, coffee.

Prohibited products:

- Carbonated drinks;
- Sugar, honey;
- Buns, bread;
- Cereals;
- **Skim** milk, kefir, yogurts;
- Margarine spreads;
- Pasta;
- Starchy vegetables;
- Candies;
- Potato chips;
- Rice;
- Potatoes;
- Breakfast cereals;
- Bread.

Eating a diet low in carbohydrates and high in fat.

1. Obligatory intake of vitamins and minerals (calcium, vitamin D, folic acid, vitamins of group B)
2. Drink water as much as possible
3. Eat products from the allowed list

It is best to consult a doctor before starting this diet because if you have a liver problem, ketogenic diet would probably not work for you.

In fact, if the body goes into ketosis, then further nutrition is very comfortable, just cook food.

Below are some options for recipes if you want a simple keto meal without frills:

Breakfast options

- Eggs and bacon
- Omelets
- Coffee with cream
- Boiled eggs with mayonnaise or butter
- Avocado, salmon and sour cream;
- Sandwiches with low-carb loaves (see the recipe below)
- Cheese with butter
- Boiled eggs, mixed with butter, chopped green onions, salt, and pepper
- A piece of brie cheese and ham
- Yogurt with high-fat content with nuts seeds and berries.

Dinner and supper

Meat, fish or chicken dishes with vegetables and fat sauce are the first thing to consider. There are many alternatives to potatoes, for example, puree from cauliflower.

Stews, soups or casseroles from low-carbohydrate ingredients are great options. Food is like science, and when you experiment it right, it will give you delicious results.

You can use most of the usual recipes, replacing or removing carbohydrate-rich foods. It is also not bad in the recipe to add fats (for example, butter, and cream). This way you can actually create healthy food recipes of your own. The best part is the experiments. While experimenting, try to make healthy fast food that will save your time and effort.

Snacks

On a low-carbohydrate diet with a lot of fat, you most likely will not want to eat often. Do not be surprised if you no longer need snacks. Many people feel great eating two or three times a day. If you need a snack, then take:

- Cheese or ham with vegetables (some people even spread butter on cheese)
- Olives
- Nuts
- Boiled egg
- Olives and nuts can replace chips. If you feel hungry between meals, you do not eat enough fat.

It is important to be proud of yourself and to achieve that you should endorse a healthy lifestyle. Ketogenic diet allows you to have a healthy lifestyle without a hassle.

Keto Bread

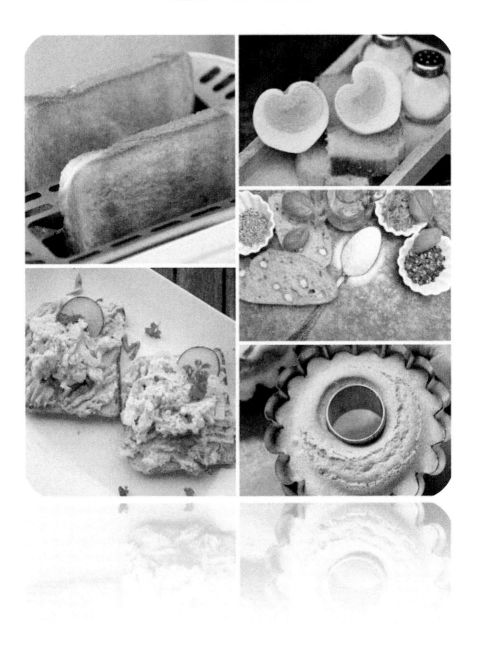

Cream Cheese Keto Bread

I genuinely enjoy consuming cream cheese, the richness of its texture and its taste makes me quite happy. This bread recipe uses cream cheese very wisely. Try it now.

Preparation Time: 10 minutes
Cooking Time: 25 minutes
Serving: 16 slices

Ingredients:
1/2 cup peanut flour
4 egg yolks
2 tablespoon erythritol
5 oz Cream Cheese
1 teaspoon Baking powder
4 tablespoon Butter
1 pinch salt

Directions:
1. Preheat the oven to 350 degrees F.
2. Combine the cream cheese with butter and mix well.
3. Add the egg yolks, salt, erythritol, and baking powder.
4. Mix well and add the peanut flour. Mix again.
5. Add to your loaf pan and bake in the oven for 25 minutes.

Nutrition Facts: (per serving)
Calories: 88 kcal | Fat: 7.5g | Carbs: 2.25g | Protein: 3.25g

Almond Coconut Bread

Combining the almond flavor and coconut flavor brings the bread to a different level. I make this for special occasions.

Preparation Time: 10 minutes
Cooking Time: 45 minutes
Serving: 20 slices

Ingredients:
2 tablespoon coconut oil
2 cup almond flour
½ teaspoon salt
½ teaspoon xanthan gum
1 teaspoon baking powder
2 eggs
½ cup melted butter

Directions:
1. Preheat oven to 355 degrees F.
2. Beat the eggs in a mixing bowl.
3. Add the butter, and coconut oil and mix well.
4. Add the baking powder, salt, xanthan gum, and almond flour.
5. Mix well and add to your loaf pan.
6. Bake in the preheated oven for 45 minutes.

Nutrition Facts: (per serving)
Calories: 234 kcal | Fat: 23g | Carbs: 1g | Protein: 7g

2 Minute Keto Bread

Are you craving for bread but you just don't want to go to the store to buy one, and you have very little time in your hand? Try this recipe and be amazed how quickly your bread can be prepared!

Preparation Time: 1 minute
Cooking Time: 1 minute
Serving: 1

Ingredients:

1 egg
1 teaspoon baking powder
1 tablespoon coconut oil
1 tablespoon coconut flour
1/3 cup almond flour
1 pinch salt
1 tablespoon sugar substitute (optional)

Directions:

7. Take a microwave safe bowl and add the egg.
8. Beat well and add the oil, flour, sugar substitute and salt.
9. Mix well and microwave for 1 minute.
10. Serve immediately.

Nutrition Facts: (per serving)

Calories: 160 kcal | Fat: 17g | Carbs: 1g | Protein: 6.5 g

Banana Bread (Keto Style)

This recipe is super healthy; it contains chia seeds, sesame seeds, and sunflower seeds. The outcome would surely amaze you.

Preparation Time: 20 minutes
Cooking Time: 45 minutes
Serving: 20 slices

Ingredients:
- ½ cup butter
- 2 tablespoon sesame seeds
- 4 drops of banana extract
- ¼ cup erythritol
- ½ teaspoon xanthium gum
- 2 tablespoon chia seeds
- 1 teaspoon baking powder
- 2 tablespoon olive oil
- 7 eggs
- 2 cups almond flour
- ½ cup sunflower seeds
- ½ teaspoon salt

Directions:
1. Preheat oven to 355 degrees F.
2. Melt the butter in a microwave.
3. Beat the eggs in a bowl until they become fluffy.
4. Add the butter, oil and beat again.

5. Add the flour, baking powder, salt, xanthium gum and sunflower seeds.
6. Mix well and add the chia seeds, erythritol and mix again.
7. Add them to the loaf pan and top with the sesame seeds.
8. Bake in the oven for about 45 minutes.

Nutrition Facts: (per serving)
Calories: 400 kcal | Fat: 37g | Carbs: 4g | Protein: 14g

Delicious Keto Bread

If you are on a keto diet and you crave for bread, what should you do? Try this basic bread recipe which is keto friendly. ☺

Preparation Time: 10 minutes
Cooking Time: 25 minutes
Serving: 20 slices

Ingredients:
1 1/2 Cup Almond Flour
3 teaspoon Baking powder
1/4 teaspoon Cream of Tartar
6 Large eggs
1 pinch salt
4 tablespoon Butter

Directions:
1. Preheat oven to 375 degrees F.
2. Melt the butter in a microwave.
3. Whisk the egg and add the cream of Tartar. Mix well.
4. Add the melted butter, baking powder, salt and almond flour. Mix well and knead into dough.
5. Add to your greased loaf pan and bake in the preheated oven for about 30 minutes.

Nutrition Facts: (per serving)
Calories: 90 kcal | Fat: 8g | Carbs: 2.25g | Protein: 4g

Keto Coconut Bread Roll

Being able to eat bread during keto diet in itself is a blessing, and when it is flavored using coconut, the joy becomes greater. ☺

Preparation Time: 10 minutes
Cooking Time: 35 minutes
Serving: 10 rolls

Ingredients:
1/2 cup Coconut flour
4 large eggs
1/2 teaspoon Baking powder
4 tablespoon Butter
2 tablespoon Psyllium Husk powder
3/4 cup Water
1 pinch salt

Directions:
1. Preheat the oven to 350 degrees F.
2. Melt the butter in a microwave.
3. Whisk the eggs in a mixing bowl.
4. Add the butter and warm water then mix well. Set aside for now.
5. Combine the coconut flour, salt, psyllium husk powder, and baking powder, salt in another bowl.
6. Add the egg mixture to the flour mixture. Knead the dough and create 10 rolls.
7. Arrange into a baking tray and let it sit for 10 minutes.

8. Bake in the oven for about 30 minutes.

Nutrition Facts: (per serving)
Calories: 102 kcal | Fat: 7g | Carbs: 5.8g | Protein: 3g

Keto Smoothies/Juices

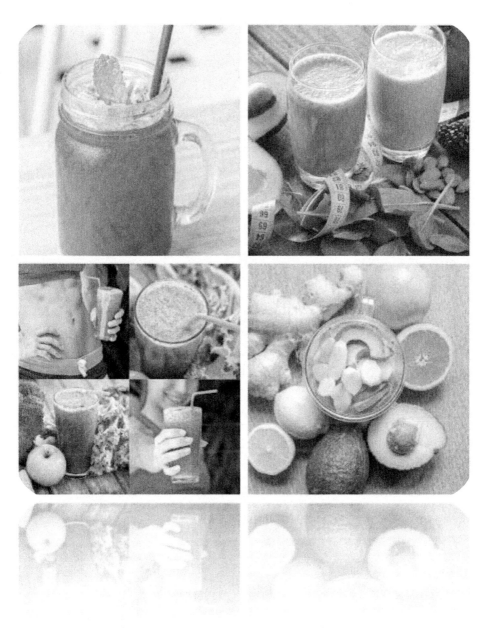

Avocado Coconut Mint Smoothie

The milky texture of coconut and avocado give this smoothie very rich texture and taste.

Preparation Time: 2 minutes
Serving: 1

Ingredients:
1/2 of an avocado, diced
5-6 large mint leaves
1/2 cup almond milk
3 sprigs of cilantro
3/4 cup full fat coconut milk
1 cup crushed ice
Sweetener to taste
1 squeeze of lime juice
1 pinch vanilla (optional)

Directions:
1. Add the coconut milk, almond milk into your food processor.
2. Add the vanilla, cilantro, lime juice, avocado, and mint.
3. Add the sweetener and crushed ice.
4. Blend until smooth and serve cold.

Nutrition Facts: (per serving)
Calories: 223g Kcal | Total Fat: 23g | Carbs: 5g | Protein: 1g

Turmeric Avocado Smoothie

This is a super smoothie containing turmeric, coconut milk, and avocado. Adding a little lime juice makes it very delicious.

Preparation Time: 2 minutes
Serving: 2

Ingredients:
1/2 avocado, diced
1 teaspoon fresh grated ginger
3/4 cup coconut milk
1/2 teaspoon turmeric
Sugar substitute to taste
1 teaspoon lemon or lime juice
1/4 cup almond milk
1 cup crushed ice
Sugar substitute (optional)

Directions:
1. In a blender, add the avocado, coconut milk, ginger and lime juice.
2. Add the almond milk, and sugar substitute.
3. Blend until smooth and add the crushed ice.
4. Blend for one more time and serve fresh.

Nutrition Facts: (per serving)
Calories: 208g kcal | Total Fat: 21g | Carbs: 5g | Protein: 1g

Raspberry Avocado Smoothie

Combining avocado and raspberry brings a very interesting flavor. Adding a little bit of lemon juice enhances the flavor.

Preparation Time: 2 minutes
Serving: 2

Ingredients:
1/2 cup raspberries
1 ripe avocado, diced
3 tablespoons lemon juice
2 tablespoons sugar substitute
1 1/3 cup water

Directions:
1. Add the diced avocado in a blender.
2. Add the lemon juice, water, and sugar substitute.
3. Blend until the mixture is perfectly smooth.

Nutrition Facts: (per serving)

Calories: 168 g kcal | Total Fat: 15g | Carbs: 8.8g | Protein: 1.5g

Strawberry Avocado Smoothie

During summer having smoothie every day becomes a routine for me... You can substitute strawberries with any other berries of your choice.

Preparation Time: 2 minutes
Serving: 3

Ingredients:
1 cup strawberries
1 tablespoon lime juice
1 avocado, diced
2 teaspoon sugar substitute
1/2 cup ice
1 1/2 cups coconut milk

Directions:
1. Add the avocado, coconut milk and lime juice in a blender.
2. Add the strawberries and ice cubes.
3. Blend until the mixture is smooth.
4. Add the sugar substitute and mix again.
5. Serve cold.

Nutrition Facts: (per serving)
Calories: 291 g kcal | Total Fat: 26.6g | Carbs: 9 g | Protein: 3.4 g

Sparkling Raspberry Limeade

Once in a while when I want to treat myself with healthy but a different beverage, this is the recipe I go for. It tastes better than the store bought Limeade.

Preparation Time: 2 minutes
Serving: 2

Ingredients:
1 Sparkling Raspberry Lemonade
2 tablespoon lime juice
1/2 cup crushed ice
1/8 teaspoon sugar substitute
1/2 cup raspberries

Directions:
1. Add the Sparkling Raspberry Lemonade in a blender.
2. Add the lime juice, raspberries, and sugar substitute.
3. Add the ice and blend until it becomes smooth.
4. Serve cold.

Nutrition Facts: (per serving)

Calories: 290 kcal | Total Fat: 0.2g | Carbs: 5.5g | Protein: 0.5g

Strawberry Limeade

Get better than store bought Limeade within just 5 minutes. The ingredients used can be easily found in your kitchen.

Preparation Time: 5 minutes

Serving: 8

Ingredients:
1 1/2 cups strawberries
1 1/2 teaspoons sugar substitute
5 ice cubes
3/4 cup fresh lime juice
5 cups water

Directions:
1. Cut the strawberries in half and add to a blender.
2. Blend until it becomes smooth.
3. Add the lime juice and blend again.
4. Transfer the mix into a pitcher.
5. Add the water and sugar substitute.
6. Add the ice cubes and mix well.
7. Serve cold.

Nutrition Facts: (per serving)

Calories: 16 | Total Fat: 0.1g | Carbs: 4.3g | Protein: 0.2g

Baked Keto Dishes

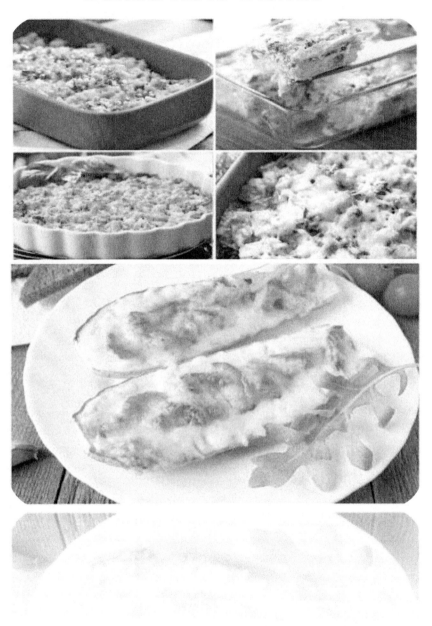

Chicken Mushroom Egg Casserole

I love casserole, and this is one dish that I never get tired of. This particular dish contains egg, chicken, and mushroom; clearly what else do you need to make it super healthy?

Preparation Time: 10 minutes
Cooking Time: 30 minutes
Serving: 6

Ingredients:
2 chicken breasts, cooked, diced
12-ounce spinach
1 ¼ cups shredded cheese, divided
¼ green bell pepper, chopped
4 mushrooms, diced
6 eggs
2 onions, chopped
1 tablespoon oil
Salt and pepper to taste
1 tablespoon heavy whipping cream
A dash of garlic powder
A dash of onion powder

Directions:
1. Preheat the oven to 350 degrees F.
2. Grease baking dish using oil.
3. In a pan add some oil and fry the onion, cooked chicken, mushroom, spinach and bell pepper for 2 minutes.
4. Add salt and pepper.

5. In a mixing bowl, beat the eggs. Add the garlic powder, onion powder, cream and cheese then mix well.
6. Add the mushroom mix into the baking dish. Pour in the egg mix on top.
7. Bake in the preheated oven for about 25 minutes.
8. Serve hot.

Nutrition Facts: (per serving)
Calories: 237 kcal | Fat: 17.7g | Carbs: 4g | Protein: 16.5g

Skinny Chicken Pesto Bake

A very simple chicken dish with a delicious basil pesto! Perfect for lunch!

Preparation Time: 10 minutes
Cooking Time: 35 minutes
Serving: 6

Ingredients:
1 tomato, sliced
2 chicken breasts
2 teaspoon grated parmesan cheese
Salt and fresh pepper to taste
4 teaspoon Skinny Basil Pesto
6 tablespoon mozzarella cheese, shredded

Directions:
1. Preheat your oven to 400 degrees F.
2. Cut the chicken into thin slices and season with salt and pepper.
3. Add parchment paper to your baking sheet.
4. Add the chicken to the baking sheet.
5. Rub the chicken using basil pesto and bake for about 15minutes.
6. Add the tomato slices and cheese and bake for another 5 minutes. Serve hot.

Nutrition Facts: (per serving)
Calories: 236 kcal | Fat: 11g | Carbs: 2.5g | Protein: 28g

Coconut Crumbled Chicken Casserole

When you do not want to eat regular casserole, try this recipe. Just adding the coconut crust makes it unique and interesting.

Preparation Time: 10 minutes
Cooking Time: 15 minutes
Serving: 3

Ingredients:
4 skinless chicken breasts
3 tablespoon desiccated coconut
2 tablespoon Thai red curry paste
300g cherry tomato
1 large aubergine, cubed
1 butternut squash, peeled, deseeded and cubed
4 tablespoon fresh breadcrumb
1 egg, beaten
1 tablespoon rapeseed oil
A handful coriander leaves, roughly chopped

Directions:
1. Preheat your oven to 475 degrees F.
2. Use cooking spray to grease your roasting tin.
3. In a bowl, combine the aubergine, butternut squash, and oil.
4. Transfer the mix into the roasting tin.
5. In another bowl, combine the coconut, salt, breadcrumbs, and pepper.

6. Beat the egg and add the chicken to it. Dip the chicken in the coconut mixture.
7. Add them to the roasting tin.
8. Add the curry paste, tomatoes and bake in the oven for nearly 12 minutes.
9. Serve hot.

Nutrition Facts: (per serving)
Calories: 276 kcal | Fat: 10.5g | Carbs: 7.7g | Protein: 26.6 g

Baked Cheesy Zucchini

Have you ever tried baked zucchini with cheese inside? Try it now; it tastes delicious.

Preparation Time: 10 minutes
Cooking Time: 50 minutes
Serving: 3

Ingredients:
4 zucchini
½ teaspoon dry basil
1 tablespoon lemon juice, fresh
Salt and pepper to taste
¼ cup parmesan
1 ½ tablespoon coconut oil

Directions:
1. Preheat the oven to 375 degrees F.
2. Add parchment paper to a baking tray.
3. Cut the stem off the zucchinis and carefully take out the flesh inside.
4. In a bowl, combine the parmesan, salt, pepper, lemon juice and basil.
5. Mix well and stuff the zucchinis using the cheese mix.
6. Add them to the baking tray.
7. Drizzle the coconut oil on top.
8. Bake in the oven for about 25 minutes. Serve hot.

Nutrition Facts: (per serving)
Calories: 45.7 kcal | Fat: 5.11g | Carbs: 4.3g | Protein: 2.24g

Low Carb Mushroom Zucchini Tofu Casserole

If you are tired of consuming beef, chicken, turkey or fish, then it is time for you to try this casserole using tofu. Tofu is a very healthy ingredient and tastes good as well.

Preparation Time: 10 minutes
Cooking Time: 1 hour
Serving: 6

Ingredients:
1 onion, chopped
2 cups chopped zucchini
1 cup mushroom
½ cup tofu, cubed
1 cup shredded cheese, divided
2 eggs
Salt and pepper to taste
1 teaspoon butter
½ cup heavy whipping cream
2 garlic cloves, mince
1 tablespoon olive oil
1/3 cup roasted chopped almonds

Directions:
1. Preheat your oven to 400 degrees F.
2. Fry the garlic, mushroom and zucchini for about 5 minutes and transfer to a bowl.
3. Add the almonds, half of the cheese, and mix well.
4. Add the tofu, and mix again.

5. Beat the eggs and cream together.
6. Add the mushroom mix into your baking dish.
7. Add the egg mix on top.
8. Top with the cheese and olive oil.
9. Bake in the oven for about 50 minutes.
10. Serve hot.

Nutrition Facts: (per serving)

Calories: 228 kcal | Fat: 19.6g | Carbs: 6.7g | Protein: 8.6g

Keto Egg Dishes

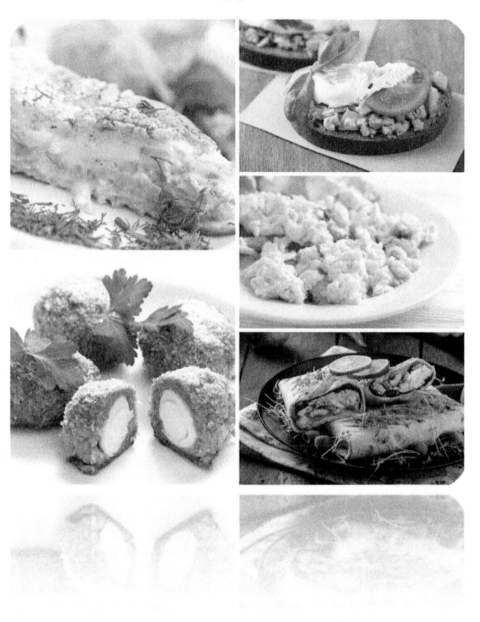

Creamy Coconut Egg Curry

Egg is a superfood and combining it with coconut milk makes it healthy. This curry is definitely something you can make for special occasions.

Preparation Time: 5 minutes
Cooking Time: 30 minutes
Servings: 12

Ingredients:
12 eggs
4 cups coconut milk
Salt to taste
2 tablespoon coconut paste
1 cup diced onion
1 tablespoon ginger garlic paste
6 green chilies
2 tablespoon olive oil

Directions

1. Hard boil the eggs with salted water (8-10 minutes).
2. Drain and get rid of the egg shells.
3. Now in a pot, add the olive oil and fry the onion for 2 minutes.
4. Add the ginger garlic paste and cook for 2 minutes.
5. Add the coconut paste and add 1 cup of milk.
6. Cover and cook for 5 minutes.
7. Add the chilies, salt, and the remaining milk.

8. Cook for 10 minutes and add the hard boiled eggs.
9. Cook for another 10 minutes and serve hot.

Nutrition Facts: (per serving)

Calories: 184 kcal | Fat: 16g | Carbs: 6.4g | Protein: 12g

Eggs Pizza

Tried sausage, chicken, pepperoni pizza? Now try this egg pizza. You would surely love it.

Preparation Time: 5 minutes
Cooking Time: 20 minutes
Servings: 4-5

Ingredients:
6 large eggs
1 1/2 teaspoon olive oil
Fresh black pepper to taste
1/4 cup vegetable broth
2 cups crushed tomatoes
1/4 teaspoon crushed red pepper
4 cloves garlic, chopped
4 basil leaves, torn
1 tablespoon chopped fresh parsley
2 tablespoon grated Pecorino Romano
Salt and fresh pepper to taste

Directions:
1. Heat the oil in a skillet, and fry the garlic for 1 minute.
2. Add the black pepper, salt, and red pepper flakes.
3. Cook for a minute and add parsley and stir.
4. Add the tomatoes and cook for another minute.
5. Add the chicken broth and cook until it comes to a boil.
6. Crack the eggs in the middle boiling mixture and add the Pecorino Romano.

7. Cover and cook for about 15 minutes.
8. Add the basil and take off the heat. Serve hot.

Nutrition Facts: (per serving)

Calories: 183 kcal | Fat: 13g | Carbs: 4.7 g | Protein: 10.3 g

Traditional Egg Mayo Salad

Egg salads are always something everyone enjoys, and this dish makes a very good side dish.

Preparation Time: 5 minutes
Cooking Time: 10 minutes
Servings: 4

Ingredients:
6 eggs
2 tablespoon mayo
2 teaspoon lemon juice
Salt to taste
Paprika to taste
Coriander to taste
1 onion, diced
Lettuce leaves to serve
½ cup chopped celery

Directions:
1. Hard boil the eggs in salted water.
2. Discard the shells and chop them finely.
3. In a bowl, add the eggs.
4. Add the mayo, lemon juice, coriander, onion, salt, celery, paprika and mix well.
5. Serve on top of lettuce leaves.

Nutrition Facts: (per serving)
Calories: 112 kcal | Fat: 7.4 g | Carbs: 1.7 g | Protein: 10g

Avocado Egg Tomato Salad

If you are up for a quick lunch, this is a healthy salad option you should go for.

Preparation Time: 5 minutes
Cooking Time: 10 minutes
Servings: 4-5

Ingredients:
6 cups spinach leaves
6 eggs
1 tomato, diced
1 onion, diced
2 avocado, diced
Cilantro to taste
Dressing:
2 tablespoon lemon juice
2 tablespoon sour cream
2 tablespoon mayo
Salt and fresh pepper to taste

Directions:
1. To make the dressing, combine all the dressing ingredients. Mix well and set aside for now.
2. Hard boil the eggs in salted water and discard the shells.
3. Chop the eggs finely and add to a bowl.
4. Add the avocado, tomatoes, onion, and cilantro.
5. Add the spinach and mix well. Finally, add the dressing and mix well.

6. Serve fresh.

Nutrition Facts: (per serving)
Calories: 264 kcal | Total fat: 21 g | Carbs: 8.5 g |
Protein: 10 g

Classic Cheesy Scotch Eggs

It is interesting how many dishes you can make using "eggs." Scotch eggs are actually classy and taste very good as well.

Preparation Time: 15 minutes
Cooking Time: 30 minutes
Servings: 8

Ingredients:
8 eggs
1 lb ground chicken
2 tablespoon mayo
2 tablespoon mustard
1 beaten egg
1 cup of low carb cheese cracker crumbs
Salt and fresh pepper to taste

Directions:
1. Start by preheating your oven to 425 degrees F.
2. Combine the cheese cracker crumbs with ground chicken.
3. Hard boil the eggs and discard the shells.
4. Use your hands and cover each egg using the chicken mix.
5. Dip each egg in the beaten egg.
6. Arrange into a baking sheet and bake for about 30 minutes.

Nutrition Facts: (per serving)
Calories: 235 kcal | Fat: 14 g | Carbs: 1.3 g | Protein: 25.6 g

Avocado Egg Crostini

Crostini is a party favorite and to make it healthy, I choose avocado and egg.

Preparation Time: 10 minutes
Cooking Time: 5 minutes
Servings: 8

Ingredients:
1 low carb loaf
3 eggs
3 tablespoon milk
Salt to taste
1 tablespoon oil
Pepper to taste
1 tablespoon butter
½ cup parmesan cheese
½ cup diced tomatoes
1 avocado
1 teaspoon lemon juice

Directions:
1. Start by preheating the oven to 350 degrees F.
2. Cut the loaf into 16 slices and arrange them into a baking sheet.
3. Add some oil on top and bake in the oven for 5 minutes.
4. In a bowl, combine the milk and eggs and mix well.
5. In a pan, melt the butter and add the egg mix.
6. Season using salt and pepper and cook until done.

7. In a bowl, mash the avocado and mix in salt and lemon juice.
8. Add the avocado mix to your toasted loaf and add the egg mix on top.
9. Add tomatoes and parmesan on top and serve.

Nutrition Facts: (per serving)

Calories: 225 kcal | Fat: 20 g | Carbs: 4.4 g | Protein: 9 g

Poached Eggs with Wild Mushroom

This is a good snacking option. Instead of consuming junk food, try this beautiful dish.

Preparation Time: 15 minutes
Cooking Time: 20 minutes
Servings: 2

Ingredients:
4 cups wild mushroom
1 tablespoon olive oil
2 garlic cloves, minced
2 eggs
Salt and pepper to taste
Hot pepper flakes to taste
Rosemary to taste
2 tablespoon chives
2 tablespoon vinegar
½ teaspoon lemon zest
2 low carb flatbreads

Directions:
1. In a skillet, heat the oil and fry the onion for 3 minutes.
2. Add the garlic, rosemary, thyme, salt, pepper flakes, mushrooms, and pepper.
3. Cook for 5 minutes and add the lemon zest, vinegar and cook for 2 minutes.
4. Toast the flatbread for 4 minutes.
5. In a pot add 2 cups of water and add a pinch of water.

6. Bring it to boil, and water-poach the eggs.
7. Serve the flatbreads with mushroom and eggs.
8. Add chives on top for garnish.

Nutrition Facts: (per serving)

Calories: 168 kcal | Fat: 8 g | Carbs: 7.4 g | Protein: 18 g

Fish

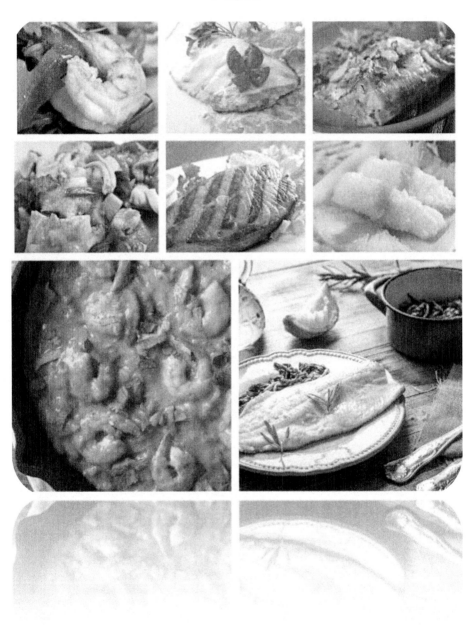

Mango Cream Sauce Sea Bass

This is a recipe that would make consuming fish fun. Anyone who doesn't like fish would also enjoy this dish. The mango sauce makes it irresistible.

Preparation Time: 10 minutes
Cooking Time: 25 minutes
Serving: 4

Ingredients:
1/2 mango, peeled
1/2 teaspoon black pepper
1 teaspoon olive oil
2 cloves minced garlic
1/2 cup chopped macadamia nuts
1/2 cup heavy cream
1 pound fresh sea bass
Salt and ground black pepper to taste
1 teaspoon lemon juice
1 pinch red pepper flakes
1 tablespoon extra-virgin olive oil
1/4 cup seasoned breadcrumbs

Directions:
1. Preheat your oven to 350 degrees F.
2. Add parchment paper to a baking sheet.
3. Combine the nuts, oil, salt, pepper, pepper flakes and bread crumbs in a blender.
4. Blend until well mixed.

5. In a pan add the mango, lemon juice, and heavy cream.
6. Bring the mixture to boil and take off the heat.
7. Fry the fish with salt and pepper and transfer to a baking tray.
8. Add the nut mix on top of the fish and bake in the oven for 10 minutes.
9. Add the mango mix and serve.

Nutrition Fats

Calories: 495 kcal | Fat: 39 g | Carb: 8.2 g | Protein: 26.7g

Baked Tilapia

This is a classic fish dish that requires very little preparation. It can be made within 30 minutes or less.

Preparation Time: 5 minutes
Cooking Time: 20 minutes
Serving: 3-4

Ingredients:
4 tilapia fillets
4 tablespoon tomato paste
2 tablespoon olive oil
Salt and pepper to taste
1 onion, sliced
4 tablespoon butter
1 teaspoon garlic powder
½ teaspoon oregano
1 bell pepper, slices

Directions:
1. Preheat your oven to 350 degrees F.
2. Use a cooking spray to grease a baking tray.
3. In a bowl, combine the salt, oil, oregano, garlic, and pepper. Mix well.
4. Coat the fish with the mixture and add to the baking tray.
5. Add the bell pepper slices and onion on top of the fish.
6. Bake for 15 minutes.

7. Add butter on top and bake for another 5 minutes.
8. Serve hot.

Nutrition Facts: (per serving)

Calories: 265 kcal | Fat: 18.4g | Carbs: 4.6g | Protein: 20.8g

Lime Flavored Mushroom Tilapia

If you want to spice up your fish dish, then try this recipe. It is a very simple dish but tastes quite good.

Preparation Time: 20 minutes
Cooking Time: 15 minutes
Serving: 2

Ingredients:
1-ounce porcini mushrooms, dried
2 limes, juiced
1 tablespoon lemon zest
Salt and pepper to taste
4-ounce tilapia fillets, halved
1 onions, chopped
2 tablespoon butter

Directions:
1. Soak the mushroom in warm water for about 20 minutes.
2. In a pan, melt the butter and sear the fish for 2 minutes.
3. Sprinkle salt and pepper on top.
4. Add the lemon juice, lemon zest and cook for 2 minutes.
5. Transfer the fish to a plate.
6. Into the same pan add the onion and mushroom.
7. Toss for about 5 minutes.
8. Serve the fish with the mushroom.

Nutrition Facts: (per serving)

Calories: 192 kcal | Fat: 8.9g | Carbs: 4.8g | Protein: 14.2g

Salmon Loaf

This is a ketogenic spin on a classic loaf dish. Adding salmon makes it super healthy.

Preparation Time: 10 minutes
Cooking Time: 45 minutes
Serving: 4

Ingredients:
2 egg, beaten
19-ounce salmon
2 tablespoon butter (melted)
½ cup milk
Salt and pepper taste
½ cup crushed saltine crackers

Directions:
1. Preheat the oven to 375 degrees F.
2. Arrange a parchment paper into a loaf pan.
3. In a mixing bowl, beat the eggs.
4. Add the butter, salt, milk, cracker, and pepper.
5. Mix well and add the salmon.
6. Mix well and add the mix to your loaf pan.
7. Bake in the oven for about 45 minutes.

Nutrition Facts: (per serving)
Calories: 332 kcal | Fat: 19g | Carbs: 3.7g | Protein: 30 g

Tomato prawn curry

Curries are so delicious and adding the tomatoes makes it even better.

Preparation Time: 10 minutes
Cooking Time: 45 minutes
Serving: 4

Ingredients:

2 cups prawns
4 teaspoon red curry paste
3 teaspoon fresh root ginger
1 cup chopped tomatoes
4 onions, chopped
2 tablespoon vegetable oil
½ cup coconut cream
Salt and pepper to taste

Directions:

1. Peel the shrimps and devein them carefully.
2. In a pot, heat the vegetable oil.
3. Fry the onion for 2 minutes and add the curry paste.
4. Add the ginger and cook for 2 minutes.
5. Add the tomatoes and cook for 5 minutes.
6. Finally, add the prawns and cook for another 2 minutes.
7. Season using salt and pepper. Serve hot.

Nutrition Facts: (per serving)
Calories: 380 kcal | Fat: 9.8 g | Carbs: 5 g | Protein: 20g

Spicy Steamed Trout

If you like spices, this is the fish dish you can try. Add a little red chili if you want your fish to be super delicious and spicy.

Preparation Time: 10 minutes
Cooking Time: 10 minutes
Serving: 4

Ingredients:
4 trout fillets
5 garlic clove, chopped
1 teaspoon lemon juice
6 baby pak choi
1 red chili, chopped
¼ teaspoon grated lime zest
4 teaspoon ginger, peeled and chopped
4 tablespoon soy sauce

Directions:
1. Arrange an aluminum foil on a plate.
2. Place the trout on it.
3. In a bowl combine the lime juice, garlic, chili, lime zest, and ginger.
4. Add on top of the fish.
5. Add the soy sauce, pak choi on it.
6. Wrap the fish and add to the trivet of your cooker.
7. Pour 1 cup of water in it and cover with lid.

8. Steam for about 10 minutes over high heat.
9. Serve hot.

Nutrition Facts: (per serving)

Calories: 399 kcal | Fat: 7g | Carbs: 4g | Protein: 29g

Cheesy Avocado Shrimp Bites

This is one snacking item that you would fall in love with. Whomever I fed, enjoyed it and wanted the recipe.

Preparation Time: 10 minutes
Cooking Time: 10 minutes
Serving: 2

Ingredients:
8 ounce cooked shrimp
3 ounce shredded cheddar cheese
1 avocado, sliced
1 pinch of garlic powder
1 tablespoon sesame oil
2 tablespoon butter
1/4 tablespoon chopped chilies
Salt and pepper to taste
1/2 cup roasted cashews
2 tortilla (low carb)

Directions:
1. Preheat the broiler.
2. Heat the oil and melt the butter in a pan.
3. Add the cashew, shrimp, chile peppers, pepper, salt and garlic powder.
4. Stir for about 3 minutes and transfer to a plate.
5. Take the tortilla and add avocado slices, the shrimp mix.
6. Add the cheese and add the tortilla into your broiler.

7. Cook for 5 minutes and serve.

Nutrition Facts: (per serving)

Calories: 305 kcal | Fat: 77.9g | Carbs: 11.7g | Protein: 22.7g

Salad

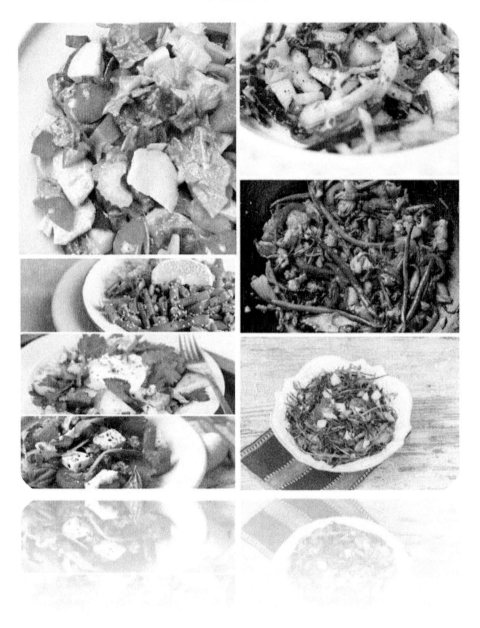

Cold Lettuce Salmon Salad

Some salads are best served cold. This particular one is one of them. You can substitute the salmon with any other fish of your choice.

Preparation Time: 10 minutes
Serving: 2

Ingredients:
1 cup boiled salmon
2 tablespoon capers
2 tablespoon plain yogurt
2 tablespoon mayo
8 lettuce leaves
Salt and pepper to taste
1 cup chopped celery

Directions:
1. Crumble the salmon in a mixing bowl.
2. Add the yogurt and mix well.
3. Add the capers, salt, celery, pepper, and mayo.
4. Mix well and finally season using salt and pepper.
5. Serve cold.

Nutrition Facts: (per serving)
Calories: 182 kcal | Fat: 7.4g | Carbs: 3.7g | Protein: 23.9g

Egg Mustard Dill pickle Salad

When you want something authentic, but it has to be healthy, this is one salad recipe you must try! It contains the flavorful mustard, dill pickle and the goodness of eggs.

Preparation Time: 10 minutes
Cooking Time: 5 minutes
Serving: 4

Ingredients:
1 head cauliflower, diced
4 eggs (hard boiled), diced
2 tablespoon chopped onion
1 tablespoon yellow mustard
½ cup mayo
Salt and pepper to taste
2 tablespoon dill pickle relish

Directions:
1. Steam the cauliflower for about 5 minutes and transfer to a mixing bowl.
2. Add the diced eggs, dill pickle relish, salt, mustard, pepper, onion and mix well.
3. Serve cold.

Nutrition Facts: (per serving)
Calories: 315 kcal | Fat: 27.5g | Carbs: 9.7g | Protein: 9.7g

Red Cabbage Shrimp with Mango Slaw

Red cabbage is perfect for the skin and body. It fights so many diseases. Incorporating it in a salad is a very good choice. I have added shrimp to make it more special.

Preparation Time: 10 minutes
Cooking Time: 10 minutes
Serving: 4

Ingredients:
1/2 head red cabbage, shredded
1 tablespoon olive oil
1 (8 oz) mango
28 extra large shrimp
1 onion, sliced into thin strips
1 teaspoon salt
1/8 ground black pepper
3/4 teaspoon turmeric
2 tablespoon fresh chopped cilantro
2 garlic cloves, crushed
1/4 teaspoon cumin
2 limes, divided
1/8 teaspoon crushed red pepper flakes

Directions:
1. In a bowl, combine the lime juice, olive oil, black pepper and 3/4 teaspoon of the salt.
2. Add the onion, cilantro, red cabbage and mango.

3. In a pan, heat some oil and fry the shrimp with garlic, turmeric, cumin, and red pepper flakes.
4. Stir for about 2 minutes and take off the heat.
5. Mix with the mango slaw.
6. Serve fresh.

Nutrition Facts: (per serving)

Calories: 228 kcal | Fat: 7g | Carbs: 10g | Protein: 25g

Asparagus Tomato Lobster Salad

This is one extravagant salad recipe that you treat yourself with after a good workout or any good news. Your guests would also enjoy it.

Preparation Time: 10 minutes
Cooking Time: 5 minutes
Serving: 2

Ingredients:
1 cup of freshly cooked lobster, chopped
2 tablespoon fresh lemon juice
1/2 cup cherry tomatoes
1/4 teaspoon salt
Black pepper, to taste
2 tablespoon diced red onion
3 1/2 cups chopped asparagus
1 basil leaf, chopped
4 teaspoons extra virgin olive oil

Directions:
1. Boil the asparagus for 3 minutes and drain well.
2. Combine the lemon juice, salt, oil, and pepper in a bowl.
3. In another bowl, combine the tomatoes, lobster, basil, asparagus, and onion.

Nutrition Facts: (per serving)
Calories: 247 kcal | Fat: 10.5g | Carbs: 14g | Protein: 27g

Avocado Romaine Tomato with Dijon Mustard Salad

This salad has a very rich dressing, which makes the salad irresistible. The avocado and grape tomatoes bring out the flavors in the salad.

Preparation Time: 10 minutes
Cooking Time: 5 minutes
Serving: 2

Ingredients:
5 cups romaine, chopped
1 onion, sliced
4 grape tomatoes
1 avocado, sliced
1 red bell pepper
Dressing
1 tablespoon minced shallots
2 tablespoon extra-virgin olive oil
1/2 teaspoon kosher salt
2 teaspoons Dijon mustard
2 tablespoon white wine vinegar
6 tablespoon 1% buttermilk
A pinch black pepper
1/4 teaspoon garlic powder

Directions:
1. In a bowl, add the dressing ingredients.
2. Mix well and set aside for now.

3. In another mixing bowl, add the onion, avocado, red bell pepper, grape tomatoes, and romaine.
4. Add the dressing on top and toss well.
5. Serve fresh.

Nutrition Facts: (per serving)

Calories: 127 kcal | Fat: 11g | Carbs: 7g | Protein: 3.5g

Avocado Chicken Blue Cheese Salad

This is another extravagant salad recipe that I make during Sundays or on special occasions. You can substitute the blue cheese with goat cheese and chicken with shrimp or tofu.

Preparation Time: 10 minutes
Cooking Time: 5 minutes
Serving: 4-5

Ingredients:
Salad
2 avocado, diced
8 cups chopped romaine lettuce
1 ½ cup cooked chicken breast, diced
6 hard-boiled eggs, diced
15 grape tomatoes, quartered
2/3 cup blue cheese

Dressing
6 tablespoon light mayonnaise
1/8 teaspoon onion powder
1/4 cup fresh chopped scallion
2/3 cup 1% buttermilk
Fresh black pepper to taste
1/8 teaspoon dried parsley
1/8 teaspoon garlic powder
1 basil leaf, chopped
Salt to taste

Directions:

1. Mix all the dressing ingredients in a mixing bowl and set aside for now.
2. In another mixing bowl, combine the avocado, romaine lettuce, chicken, eggs, and tomatoes.
3. Mix well and add the blue cheese.
4. Add the dressing and toss everything well together.
5. Serve fresh.

Nutrition Facts: (per serving)

Calories: 368 kcal | Fat: 21g | Carbs: 7,8g | Protein: 32g

Pear Red Cabbage Chicken Salad

Incorporating fruits into your salad is not always a terrible idea, in fact adding fruit can even uplift the taste of the salad. This is one such salad, the sweetness of the pear make it very flavorful.

Preparation Time: 10 minutes
Serving: 4

Ingredients:
1 large pear, sliced
2 tablespoons extra-virgin olive oil
Pinch of salt
Black pepper to taste
2 cups chopped chicken breast, cooked
2 celery stalks, thinly sliced on the bias
1 cup red cabbage, shredded
1 tablespoon sugar substitute
¾ cup cheese, crumbled
8 butter lettuce leaves
2 tablespoons apple cider vinegar
¼ cup chopped fresh parsley leaves

Directions:
1. Combine the sugar substitute, oil, salt, vinegar, and pepper.
2. Mix well and add the cabbage, celery, pear and parsley.
3. Toss nicely and add the vinegar mixture.
4. Toss again and refrigerate for 1 hour.

5. Arrange the lettuce leaves into a serving dish.
6. Add butter on top of the lettuce leaves.
7. Add the chicken mixture and serve.

Nutrition Facts: (per serving)
Calories: 341 kcal | Fat: 18g | Carbs: 12g | Protein: 27g

Avocado Jalapeno Tomato Jumbo Shrimp Salad

I love avocado and incorporating it in my daily meals gives me and my tummy a relief.
It is one such superfood that you cannot get enough of.

Preparation Time: 10 minutes
Serving: 2

Ingredients:
1/4 cup chopped red onion
1 jalapeno, diced
2 limes, juice of
Black pepper to taste
1 lb jumbo shrimp cooked
1 tomato, diced
1/4 teaspoon salt
1 avocado, diced
1 tablespoon chopped cilantro
1 teaspoon olive oil

Directions:
1. Combine the onion, oil, salt, lime juice, and pepper in a mixing bowl.
2. In another bowl, combine the avocado, shrimp, jalapeño, and tomatoes.
3. Mix well and add the cilantro, and add some more seasoning if needed. Serve fresh.

Nutrition Facts: (per serving)
Calories: 197 kcal | Fat: 8g | Carbs: 7g | Protein: 25g

Coconut Chicken Bean salad

Have you ever tried coconut dressing in your salad? This is not just another boring salad dressing. Your salad would surely taste better when you add this dressing on top.

Preparation Time: 10 minutes
Cooking Time: 5 minutes
Serving: 4

Ingredients:
4 cooked, skinless chicken breasts
400g runner beans, sliced
1/3 teaspoon ginger powder
4 shallots, finely sliced
A small bunch mint leaves
½ teaspoon coriander
1 lemongrass, finely sliced
Coconut dressing
3 bird's eye chili, finely diced
5 tablespoon fish sauce
2 teaspoon lime juice
350ml coconut cream
3 garlic clove, crushed

Directions:
1. In a bowl, combine the bird's eye chili, fish sauce, lime juice, coconut cream, and garlic.
2. Mix well and set aside for now.

3. In a pot, cook the beans with water for about 5 minutes.
4. Drain and rinse well. Transfer to a mixing bowl.
5. Add the shallots, herbs, ginger, and chicken.
6. Add the coconut mixture and toss well.
7. Serve fresh.

Nutrition Facts: (per serving)
Calories: 425 kcal | Fat: 11g | Carbs: 6g | Protein: 23g

Soup

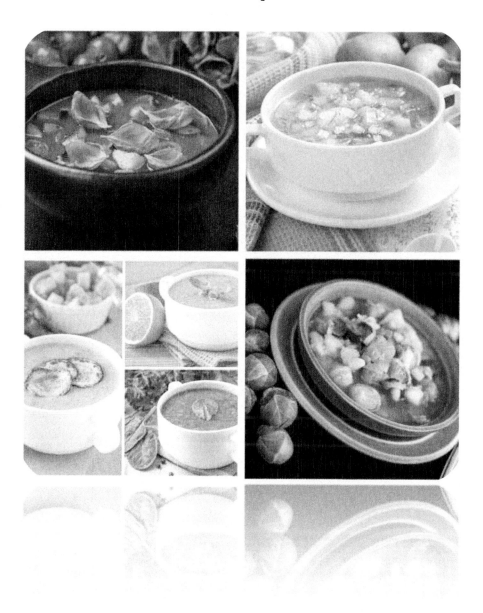

Tomato Carrot Basil Soup

Soups are the perfect comfort food, and it is even better when you can have it within 30 minutes.

Preparation Time: 10 minutes
Cooking Time: 25 minutes
Serving: 6

Ingredients:
2 teaspoons olive oil
1 cup diced celery
1 cup diced carrots
1/2 cup diced onions
2 tablespoons low carb flour
1/3 cup grated Pecorino Romano cheese
3 1/2 cups chicken broth
1 3/4 cups milk
1 tablespoon unsalted butter
2 cups diced tomatoes
1 sprig fresh thyme
1/4 cup fresh basil, chopped
2 bay leaves
3/4 teaspoon salt
Fresh black pepper, to taste

Directions:
1. In a pressure cooker, add the oil, butter, carrots, celery, and onion.

2. Stir for 5 minutes and add the flour, milk, broth, and tomatoes.
3. Add the bay leaves, basil, thyme, salt, and pepper.
4. Cover and cook on high heat for 10 minutes.
5. Add the cheese and cook for another minute.
6. Serve hot.

Nutrition Facts: (per serving)

Calories: 230 kcal | Fat: 15.7 g | Carbs: 11g | Protein: 10.6g

Chicken Cabbage Soup

When I am tired of boring soups, I try this recipe; the ground chicken makes it very delicious and flavorful. I have used green cabbage, but red cabbage can be used here as well.

Preparation Time: 10 minutes
Cooking Time: 25 minutes
Serving: 7

Ingredients:
1 lb ground chicken
4 cups chicken stock
2 cups diced tomatoes
5 cups chopped green cabbage
1 1/2 teaspoon salt
1/2 cup diced celery
1/2 cup diced carrot
1/2 cup diced onion
2 bay leaves

Directions:
1. In a pressure cooker add the carrot, chicken, tomatoes, cabbage, onion, salt, celery, and stock.
2. Mix well and cover with the lid.
3. Cook on high heat for about 20 minutes.
4. Serve hot.

Nutrition Facts: (per serving)
Calories: 123 kcal | Fat: 3.6g | Carbs: 7.4g | Protein: 19.4g

Brussels Sprouts Soup

When you know you need to eat healthily but you want to have a tasty meal as well, this is the soup recipe you should go for. The roasted technique adds the flavor here.

Preparation Time: 10 minutes
Cooking Time: 25 minutes
Serving: 6

Ingredients:

Canola cooking spray
16 oz cauliflower florets
Black pepper, to taste
16 oz brussels sprouts
3 1/2 cups vegetable broth
1/2 cup chopped shallots
1 teaspoon butter
2 tablespoon olive oil
3/4 teaspoon salt

Directions:

1. Preheat your oven to 450 degrees F.
2. Add aluminum foil to your baking sheet.
3. Add the Brussels sprout and cauliflower to it.
4. Bake in the oven for 25 minutes.
5. In a pan, melt the butter and fry the shallots for 3 minutes.
6. Pour in broth and cook until it comes to boil.
7. Add all the ingredients in the skillet.

8. Cover and cook for 10 minutes on high heat.
9. Add the roasted vegetables and cook for 2 more minutes.
10. Serve hot.

Nutrition Facts: (per serving)
Calories: 173 kcal | Fat: 8g | Carbs: 10.2g | Protein: 6.5g

Creamy Cauliflower Soup

I love cauliflower soup, and my version is so creamy with butter and heavy cream that no one can resist it.

Preparation Time: 10 minutes
Cooking Time: 1 hour
Serving: 6

Ingredients:
8 cups vegetable broth
1 cup heavy cream
3 tablespoon butter
2 tablespoon olive oil
3 garlic cloves
3 leeks, diced
Salt and pepper to taste
1 cauliflower heat, chopped

Directions:
1. In a pressure cooker, add the butter and oil and let it melt.
2. Add the garlic, leek, and cauliflower.
3. Cook for 2 minutes and pour in the broth.
4. Cover and cook for 10 minutes on high heat. Use a hand blender to blend.
5. Season with salt, pepper and add the heavy cream.
6. Mix well and serve hot.

Nutrition Facts: (per serving)
Calories: 155 kcal | Fat: 13.1g | Carbs: 8.3g | Protein: 2.4g

Cheesy Broccoli Soup

Broccoli is a super food, and you just cannot have enough of it. We should try to eat this green vegetable as much as possible. If you do not like it steamed, or stir-fried, try this recipe. It is really delicious.

Preparation Time: 10 minutes
Cooking Time: 25 minutes
Serving: 7

Ingredients:
¼ cup shredded cheddar cheese
1 onion, chopped
2 pounds broccoli, chopped
5 cups vegetable broth
1 tablespoon olive oil
Salt and pepper to taste
2 garlic cloves, mince
¼ cup lemon juice

Directions:
1. Take a pressure cooker and fry the onion, garlic in oil for 2 minutes.
2. Add in the broccoli.
3. Use salt and pepper to season
4. Stir well and pour the broth.
5. Cover and cook on high flame for 5 minutes.
6. Add the lemon juice and use a hand blender to blend.
7. Serve hot with cheese on top.

Nutrition Facts: (per serving)
Calories: 97 kcal | Fat: 3.6g | Carbs: 13g | Protein: 5g

Stew

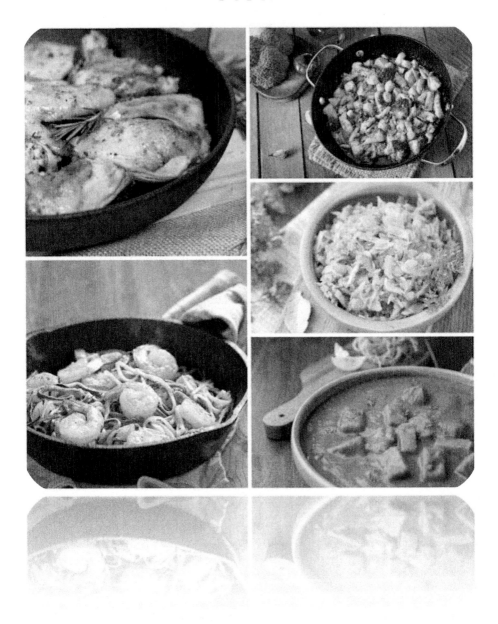

Low Carb Chicken Zucchini Shrimp Stew

I love stew! I have made this so many times and relished it with pleasure each time.

Preparation Time: 10 minutes
Cooking Time: 25 minutes
Serving: 8

Ingredients:
1 pound cooked chicken breasts, diced
2 zucchinis, chopped
1 can crushed tomatoes
1 onion, chopped
1 pound cooked shrimp
1 tablespoon butter
1 teaspoon hot sauce
3 green bell pepper, diced
1 tablespoon olive oil
6 garlic cloves, mince
1 cup chicken broth

Directions:
1. Heat the olive oil in a skillet and melt the butter.
2. Add the garlic, onion, and stir for 3 minutes.
3. Add the rest of the ingredients except the shrimp and chicken.
4. Cover and bring it to boil.
5. Simmer for about 10 minutes.
6. Add the shrimp and chicken to the skillet.

7. Cover and cook for another 2-3 minutes.

Nutrition Facts: (per serving)

Calories: 220.5 kcal | Fat: 9.5g | Carbs: 7.5g | Protein: 25.8g

Low Carb Chicken Tomato Tofu Stew

This is another stew recipe that contains the richness of tofu. You can substitute the ground chicken with mushroom if you like. The stew is filled with tomato flavor.

Preparation Time: 10 minutes
Cooking Time: 25 minutes
Serving: 2-3

Ingredients:

½ pound lean ground chicken
1 cup diced tomatoes
1 teaspoon oil
½ cup tofu, diced
1 cup tomato sauce
3 celery stalks, chopped
½ onion, chopped

Directions:

1. In a pressure cooker, add the oil, chicken, and stir for 5 minutes.
2. Add the onion, diced tomatoes, tofu, tomato sauce and celery.
3. Stir well and cover with lid.
4. Cook for about 20 minutes. Serve hot.

Nutrition Facts: (per serving)
Calories: 178 kcal | Fat: 8.5 g | Carbs: 7 g | Protein: 18.8g

Chicken Cabbage Stew

When you know you want to stay healthy but eat deliciously, this is the stew you should try. It is simple and delicious.

Preparation Time: 20 minutes
Cooking Time: 1 hour
Serving: 8

Ingredients:
8-ounce plum tomatoes, chopped
1 1/3 cups hot chicken broth
2 pounds chicken
1 teaspoon Greek seasoning
8-ounce tomato sauce
¼ cup chopped celery
2 bay leaves
8 ounce shredded cabbage
1 cube chicken bouillon
Salt and pepper to taste
2 onions, chopped

Directions:
1. In a skillet, fry the chicken for 3 minutes.
2. Transfer the chicken to a bowl and add the chicken bouillon.
3. Add the onion, bay leaves, salt, black pepper and Greek seasoning.
4. Return the mixture to the skillet.
5. Add the broth, and cover with lid.

6. Cook for 20 minutes and add the remaining ingredients.
7. Cook for another 15 minutes.
8. Serve hot.

Nutrition Facts: (per serving)

Calories: 372 kcal | Fat: 22.7g | Carbs: 8 g | Protein: 31.8g

Chicken Onion with Mushroom

This curry takes less than an hour to prepare and tastes quite good. It is perfect for a lazy dinner.

Preparation Time: 20 minutes
Cooking Time: 40 minutes
Serving: 4

Ingredients:
8 oz sliced mushrooms
1 onion, sliced
1/2 lb chicken, thinly sliced
Garlic powder to taste
1/2 teaspoon olive oil
Salt to taste
2 cups of water
Pepper to taste

Directions:
1. Season the chicken slices using salt, pepper and garlic powder.
2. In a skillet, sear the chicken slices for 2 minutes and transfer to a dish.
3. Add the onion, mushroom, and salt. Toss for about 2 minutes and return the chicken to the skillet.
4. Pour in water and cover with lid. Cook for 20 minutes on medium-high heat. Serve hot.

Nutrition Facts: (per serving)
Calories: 96 kcal | Fat: 4.1g | Carbs: 3.5g | Protein: 12.8g

Garlic Oregano Chiptole Chicken Stew

When you are tired of regular stews and curries, this is the dish you should opt for. It contains oregano, chipotles in adobo sauce, bay leaves which adds so much flavor in the stew.

Preparation Time: 20 minutes
Cooking Time: 40 minutes
Serving: 8

Ingredients:
3 lbs chicken
5 cloves garlic
1 tablespoon ground oregano
1 lime, juice
2 1/2 teaspoons salt
Black pepper to taste
1 tablespoon ground cumin
1/2 onion, diced
2-4 tablespoon chipotles in adobo sauce
3 bay leaves
1 cup water
1 teaspoon olive oil

Directions:
1. In a blender, add the cumin, garlic, oregano, onion, lime juice, chipotles, and water.
2. Blend until smooth. Cut the chicken into pieces.
3. Season the chicken using salt and pepper.
4. Sear the chicken in a skillet from both sides.

5. Now transfer the chicken into a pressure cooker. Add the lime juice mixture.

6. Cover with lid. Cook for about 20 minutes on high heat.
7. Use a fork to shred the chicken and again cook for 10 minutes.
8. Serve hot.

Nutrition Facts: (per serving)

Calories: 153 kcal | Fat: 4.5g | Carbs: 2g | Protein: 24g

Shopping List

Meat

10 lb chicken

Seafood

2 lb shrimp

2 lb Salmon

2 lb tilapia

2 lb trout

1 lb lobster

Vegetable

½ lb onion

4 Cauliflowers

1 can sugar snap peas

Collard Greens

2 Broccolis

Grape tomatoes

2 lb bell pepper

Tomatoes

Zucchini

Chilies

Fruits

Strawberries

Pear

Mango

Dairy

2-liter coconut milk

1 cup blue cheese

1 packet heavy cream

1 packet goat cheese

1-liter milk

2 lb cream cheese

Ketogenic Butter

1lb mozzarella cheese

Condiments

1 bottle ketchup

Coconut oil

Olive oil

Vanilla extract

Coconut extract

Nuts

1 packet Almond

Other

Ketogenic sugar substitute
Tofu
24 eggs
psyllium husk powder
Xanthun Gum
2 lb mushroom
Cream of Tartar
Baking powder

Flour
Almond flour
Coconut flour
Peanut flour

Herbs
Thyme
Rosemary
Parsley
Italian Herbs
Oregano

Spices
Salt
Sesame seeds
Black pepper
Baking powder
Garlic powder

Printed in Great Britain
by Amazon

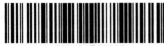

76008429R00058